Sex and health:

VARIOUS WAYS TO ENJOY INTERCOURSE

By

Elizabeth C. Barb

Tablet of contents

Introduction

Chapter 1: The Connection Between Sexuality and Health

Given the frequent and close connections between these two facets of life, it is crucial to take into account the link between health and sex. This chapter will examine the connections between physical and sexual health as well as the potential effects of sexual conduct on general health.
We'll also go over how crucial it is for couples to communicate about issues related to their reproductive health.

Chapter 2: Understanding Sexual Health

A wide variety of factors, including the physical, emotional, and social facets of sexuality, are included in the complex and multifaceted notion of sexual health. This chapter will examine the definition of healthy sexual functioning as well as the ways that different medical conditions may affect sexual health. We'll also talk about how important it is to spread information about appropriate sexual conduct.

Common sexual health issues in Chapter 3

Individuals may experience a range of reproductive health issues over the course of their lives. The most prevalent sexual health issues, such as STDs, sexual dysfunction, and problems with sexual orientation and gender identification, will be discussed in this chapter. We will also go over how to handle and address these issues.

Chapter 4: Preserving Sexual Wellness and Health

Taking care of both the physical and emotional facets of sexuality is necessary for maintaining sexual health and well-being. In this chapter, we'll look at some tactics for fostering healthy sexual behavior, such as empowering sexuality beliefs, engaging in safe sex, and looking for supportive partnerships. We will also go over the value of routine exams and tests for preserving sexual health.

Chapter 5: Navigating Sexual Health in Relationships

For people in relationships, whether they are just getting started or have been together for a while, sexual wellness is a crucial factor. In this last chapter, we'll look at some of the opportunities and problems that can emerge when it comes to relationships and sexual health. We will go over the value of open conversation between partners regarding issues related to sexual health as well as methods for continuing healthy sexual habits. Finally, we'll look at how people can speak up for their own sexual health needs and try to build relationships that are respectful and helpful.

Chapter 1: The Relationship between Sexuality and Health

Since both play significant parts in one's physical, psychological, and emotional well-being, health and sex are inextricably linked. One way to describe the connection between sex and health is as a multifaceted one, with many different factors affecting one another. While having a fulfilling sex life can improve both physical and emotional health, having a sexual life that is unhealthy can have the opposite effect. In this essay, the complicated connection between health and sex will be examined. The effects that each can have on the other will be discussed, as well as some methods that people can employ to keep both their health and their sexual lives fulfilling.

One of the most important variables that can affect sexual function and satisfaction is physical health. Sexual arousal and function problems can be brought on by certain medical conditions, including diabetes, hypertension, and heart disease. These ailments may harm the nerves or blood vessels, which may restrict blood supply to the genitalia or lessen sensation. Drugs that are prescribed to address these conditions, such as blood pressure medications, hormone therapies, and antidepressants, can make sexual issues worse, such as low libido or trouble eliciting an orgasm.

Contrarily, regular sexual exercise can have a variety of physical advantages. Since it can raise heart rate, blood flow, and oxygenation of the body, sexual activity is frequently hailed as a fantastic type of cardiovascular exercise. Endorphins are naturally occurring chemicals that provide pain relief, pleasure, and relaxation. Sexual action can trigger their release. The immune system can also be strengthened by sexual exercise by increasing the production of antibodies that ward off illnesses and infections.The connection between sex and mental wellness is also complicated. Sexual function can be negatively impacted by psychological stress, depression, anxiety, or trauma, which can result in decreased libido, trouble getting an erection or orgasm, and decreased sexual satisfaction. Low self-esteem or a negative body image can also affect a person's sexual confidence and desire, which can make them reluctant or uncomfortable during sexual interactions. On the other hand, having a fulfilling and enjoyable sexual relationship can also be beneficial for mental health.

Enhancing self-esteem and body image, as well as lowering tension and anxiety, can all result from sexual intimacy.

A crucial component of the connection between health and sex is sexual wellness. According to the World Health Organization, sexual health is "a state of physical, emotional, mental, and social well-being in relation to sexuality." A positive and respectful view of sexuality, the capacity to speak effectively about sexual matters, and the knowledge and ability to participate in safe and consensual sexual behavior are all aspects of sexual health that go beyond the absence of disease or dysfunction.

STIs, unintended pregnancies, and sexual disorders are just a few of the manifestations of poor sexual health. STIs have the potential to lead to serious and protracted health problems, such as infertility, pelvic inflammatory disease, and chronic discomfort. Unwanted pregnancy can cause mental distress and have negative effects on one's health, such as unsafe abortion or labor complications. Sexual dysfunction can affect sexual pleasure and can be a sign of underlying health issues, such as erectile dysfunction or premature ejaculation.

Effective contraception, routine STI testing, and open conversation with sexual partners about sexual health and behavior are all part of maintaining good sexual health. STIs and unintended pregnancies can be prevented by using condoms during safe intercourse and practicing contraception. A more fulfilling and satisfying sexual experience can be had by having open and honest communication with one's sexual partners. This will help to improve trust and understanding of one another's wants and desires.

Despite the complex connection between health and sex, there are a number of lifestyle changes people can make to improve their general well-being as well as their sexual function and happiness. Adopting healthy habits can enhance physical and emotional health, resulting in an increase in energy and vitality.

These habits include regular exercise, a balanced diet, and enough sleep. By lowering anxiety and fostering relaxation, practicing relaxation methods like yoga or meditation can help improve sexual function.
The function and enjoyment of sexual activity can also be improved by the use of sexual aids like lubricants or sex toys. Sex toys can spice up and add novelty to sexual encounters, while lubricants can help with dryness or discomfort during sex. To address sexual dysfunction, communication issues, or other sexual health issues, consulting a doctor or other expert in the field of sexual health can be helpful.

In summation, there are many different ways in which health and sex are related. Sexual, mental, and physical health can all have a significant effect on one another and on general well-being. Adopting healthy habits, engaging in safe sexual activity, effectively communicating with sexual partners, and seeking expert assistance when necessary are all methods for promoting good health and sexual pleasure. People can have satisfying and enjoyable sex lives that improve their overall sense of health and happiness by actively pursuing their sexual and physical well-being.

Chapter 2: Understanding Sexual Health

A condition of physical, emotional, mental, and social well-being with regard to sexuality is referred to as sexual health. It covers a wide variety of elements that affect a person's overall sexual well-being, such as healthy relationships, reproductive health, and the avoidance of STDs and other diseases.

Knowledge of Sexual Health

One of the most important elements of overall health and well-being is sexual health, which has many different facets. However, taking into account the subjectivity of sexuality, it is not just limited to the physical element. Sexuality also affects a person's emotional and spiritual well-being. As a result, sexual health is a wide concept that encompasses physical, mental, and social well-being in addition to the absence of diseases or infections. We must research some of its aspects in order to better comprehend sexual wellness.

Physical Fitness

Physical health is one of the most important aspects of reproductive health. The physical side of sexuality, such as the reproductive system's normal operation and structure, is the emphasis on physical health. It also involves avoiding unintended pregnancy and being free of STIs (sexually transmitted infections).

Infections Transmitted Sexually

Sexual contact with an infected person is the primary method of transmission for STIs, a collection of contagious diseases. With one million new infections occurring daily throughout the globe, STIs are a serious public health issue. HIV/AIDS, herpes simplex virus, chlamydia, gonorrhea, human papillomavirus (HPV), and syphilis are a few examples of prevalent STIs.

People must be proactive and take the appropriate precautions to avoid STIs. Using barriers during sexual contacts, such as condoms, dental dams, and gloves, is the most efficient method to prevent STIs. Regular testing is also required for spotting STIs early and seeking the appropriate care.

Reproductive Fitness

Another crucial component of sexual health is reproductive health, which is concerned with the condition and health of the reproductive system. Men and women can engage in secure and satisfying sexual activities without running the risk of unintended pregnancy, infertility, or other health issues thanks to reproductive health.

Not only does preventing unintended pregnancies benefit a person's general sexual health, but it also has social and economic ramifications. The use of contraception is the most efficient way to avoid unintended pregnancies. Oral contraceptive pills, condoms, intrauterine devices, vaginal rings, injections, and patches are just a few of the contraceptive options accessible.

Mental Wellness

Mental health, which is concerned with a person's psychological and emotional well-being in relation to their sexual encounters, is also a part of sexual health. By enhancing one's self-esteem and fostering feelings of pleasure and fulfillment, healthy sexual experiences can considerably improve one's mental health.

On the other hand, not all sexual experiences are beneficial, and some may be detrimental to a person's emotional health. An individual's quality of life may be negatively impacted by feelings of guilt, humiliation, and anxiety brought on by sexual abuse, trauma, and assault. Individuals who go through such experiences need expert assistance to cope and manage their emotions.

Social Welfare

The societal aspect of sexual health is concerned with how society perceives sexuality and the effects that stigma, prejudice, and inequality have on people. A community that embraces sexual diversity, encourages healthy relationships and eradicates harmful cultural practices is what sexual health seeks to achieve.

Education's Function

Ending stigmatization and encouraging healthy sexual behaviors both require education. By providing them with information about sexual health, including topics like contraception, STIs, safe sex, healthy relationship traits, and consent, appropriate sexual education can empower individuals.

Not just for children, sexual education is crucial for adults as well. Adults can gain from sexual education because it gives them access to resources for reproductive health and provides knowledge about consent that will help them avoid unwanted sexual experiences. The best teaching strategies are careful because they primarily concentrate on age; they are created to be age-specific, giving the degree of knowledge that satisfies questions within that age range, but they also grow together.

Conclusion

More than just the physical side of sexuality is involved in sexual wellness. It covers a range of areas, such as social, emotional, and bodily well-being. In order to encourage healthy sexual behavior, positive interactions, and the prevention of STIs and other diseases, it is crucial to understand sexual health. To stay current on the most recent knowledge and enhance the general sexual health of people and society, it is crucial to engage in ongoing sexual education.

Chapter 3: Typical Sexual Health Issues

One's overall health and well-being, particularly sexual health, are essential. It covers a wide variety of topics, including keeping healthy sexual relationships and preventing sexually transmitted infections (STIs). Despite the significance of reproductive health, many people are still reluctant to talk about their worries or ask for assistance when they run into issues. The common sexual health issues individuals encounter will be covered in this book, along with solutions. STIs are a significant concern for those who engage in sexual activity. STIs come in a wide variety of forms, from comparatively innocuous conditions like genital warts to fatal illnesses like HIV/AIDS. Using condoms while engaging in sexual activity is the best method to stop the spread of STIs. The majority of STIs can be successfully avoided by using condoms, and they also help avoid unintended pregnancy. Even with appropriate use, condoms are not 100% effective, so there is a chance of getting an STI. Regular STI testing is also crucial, particularly for those who engage in multiple sexual relationships or don't consistently use condoms. STI testing can aid in the early detection of infections and enable prompt therapy.

Erectile dysfunction (ED) is a further prevalent issue with sexual health. (ED). The inability of a man to sustain an erection during sexual activity is known as ED. Physical, psychological, or a mix of the two may be to blame for this. Diabetes, heart illness, and the adverse effects of some medications are examples of physical causes of ED. Anxiety, depression, and worry are psychological elements that can influence ED. The underlying reason for ED can influence the type of treatment needed. Medication or surgery might be required for physical causes. It may be suggested to seek counseling or therapy for psychological reasons. Exercise, weight loss, and other lifestyle modifications can also help avoid or reduce the symptoms of ED.

Another typical issue with sexual health is low libido or sexual urge. A decrease in libido is thought to occur in about 30% of women and 15% of men at some time in their lives. Hormonal disorders, worry, problems in relationships, depression, and illnesses like diabetes and thyroid disorders can all contribute to low libido.

The underlying reason for low libido affects the course of treatment. For menopausal women, hormone replacement treatment (HRT) may be advised. Counseling or therapy may be beneficial for dealing with psychological or relationship problems. A change in lifestyle, such as regular exercise and stress management methods, can also help libido.

Men, particularly younger men, frequently worry about their sexual health when they experience premature ejaculation (PE). PE is characterized by excessive ejaculation during intercourse, typically within two minutes of penetration. PE can be brought on by both physical (such as low testosterone levels) and psychological (such as worry and anxiety) factors. Depending on the underlying reason, PE treatment can change. While medication or HRT may be suggested for physical causes, counseling or therapy can be useful in addressing psychological factors.

Another problem with sexual health that many people experience, particularly women, is pain during intercourse. Numerous conditions, such as infections, hormonal imbalances, and psychological problems, can result in pain during intercourse. The underlying reason determines the course of treatment. Antibiotics or antifungal medications may be necessary for infections. HRT can be used to address hormonal imbalances, while therapy or counseling may be necessary for psychological issues. Lubrication can also be useful for lessening sex-related discomfort.

Another typical issue with sexual health that can impact both men and women is sexual dysfunction. Sexual dysfunction is any ongoing issue that makes engaging in sexual action challenging, uncomfortable, or unpleasant. Physical or psychological variables, such as hormonal imbalances, anxiety, melancholy, and relationship problems, can contribute to sexual dysfunction. The underlying reason for sexual dysfunction affects the course of treatment. Surgery or drugs might be required in some circumstances.

Addressing psychological issues may benefit from counseling or therapy, as well as lifestyle modifications like frequent exercise and stress-reduction methods.

In summary, sexual health is a crucial component of general health and well-being. STIs, erectile dysfunction, low libido, early ejaculation, pain during intercourse, and sexual dysfunction are some common sexual health issues. Depending on the root reason, these issues may be treated with medication, therapy, or lifestyle changes. It is crucial for people with sexual health issues to get assistance and guidance from medical experts. Maintaining healthy sexual relationships and preventing the spread of STIs also require an open dialogue with one's sexual partners.

Chapter 4: Preserving Sexual Wellness and Health

One of the most important aspects of maintaining general health and well-being is sexual health and wellness. The World Health

Organization (WHO) defines sexual health as "a state of physical, emotional, mental and social well-being in relation to sexuality," whereas sexual wellness is a comprehensive strategy for improving sexual health through open and honest communication, self-care, and positive sexual experiences. We shall examine numerous strategies for preserving sexual health and wellness in this essay.

1. Engaging in Safe Sex

The practice of safe sex is one of the most crucial aspects of preserving sexual health and wellness. This calls for the use of protection during sexual activity, such as condoms, dental dams, or other barrier techniques. Sexually transmitted diseases (STIs), unintended pregnancies, and any other possible risks connected with sexual activity are all prevented via safe sex. It's crucial to talk about, clarify, and set expectations with sexual partners. Safe sexual practices can also help people feel calmer and less stressed.

2. Interaction

Maintaining sexual fitness and health requires effective communication. An individual can be empowered to enjoy sexual encounters without feeling guilty or ashamed by having an open and honest conversations with sexual partners about their emotional and physical needs, boundaries, and expectations. This is crucial for people who have had sexual trauma or who are struggling with mental health issues.

Maintaining sexual health also requires communication with medical professionals. Potential health risks can be identified and prevented through routine check-ups, testing for STIs and other diseases, and discussing any worries or changes in sexual behavior. Finding the best course of action for each client might be aided by candidly discussing any sexual health concerns with providers.

3. Self-Care

Self-care routines can improve sexual fitness and health. Regular exercise, a good diet, getting enough sleep, and stress management are a few examples of these habits. Exercises like meditation, yoga, and mindfulness can enhance mental and emotional well-being, which in turn can enhance sexual health.

Sexual health maintenance also requires maintaining adequate cleanliness. Sexual health can be adversely affected by infections and abnormalities, which can be avoided by practicing proper personal cleanliness. For optimum sexual health, regular bathing, wearing clean clothing and underwear, and good genital cleanliness is necessary.

4. Refraining from Dangerous or Harmful Behaviors

Sexual wellness and sexual health can suffer if unsafe or dangerous sexual behavior is engaged in. Unprotected intercourse, taking part in risky activities like sharing needles, or having sex while intoxicated are a few examples of these practices. The risk of STIs, unintended pregnancies, and other potential health problems can be decreased by refraining from these habits.

5. Self-education

Maintaining long-term sexual health requires education about sexual health and wellness. Learning about various forms of contraception, STIs, and the value of personal boundaries may be part of this. Learning more about one's own body, desires, and preferences with regard to sex can also be beneficial to one's sexual health.

People should conduct studies to gain a deeper knowledge of the complexity of sexual behavior and how it is related to health problems. Insights into the complicated symptoms, diseases, and the most effective approaches can be gained by looking for materials, workshops, open discussions, and other educational opportunities.

6. Seeking Assistance

In order to preserve sexual well-being and health, it can be helpful for people to seek support. Support can come from a variety of sources, including close friends, family, or medical experts. Finding support can offer a secure setting to talk about sexual health issues and locate services, such as therapists or specialized programs.

7. Using Consent.

In order to sustain sexual health and wellness, consent is essential. Respecting one's own preferences and confirming that both partners have provided "affirmative consent" to engaging in sexual activity are essential components of practicing consent. This entails making every effort to prevent scenarios in which the spouse might feel forced or coerced. People should, when appropriate, seek affirmative consent and make sure that their views are valued and accepted.

8. Making use of the Proper Items

In order to preserve sexual health and wellness, it can be helpful to use the right goods for sexual activities. These goods could be lubricants, condoms, or other types of barrier defense. There are numerous organic and natural products available today that can increase enjoyment while yet emphasizing safety.

Finally, preserving sexual health and wellness is essential to advancing general health and well-being. To achieve this, one must establish good personal hygiene habits, communicate clearly with sexual partners and healthcare professionals, abstain from dangerous or harmful behaviors, and actively seek support when required. Sexual health and wellness can be improved further by practicing self-care, learning more about sexual health, practicing consent, and utilizing the right products. In the end, preserving sexual health and wellness can result in a more rewarding and joyful sexual experience.

Chapter 5: Navigating Sexual Health in Relationships

Any relationship should place a high priority on sexual health because it is an essential part of overall health and well-being. Despite its significance, maintaining sexual health in relationships can be difficult for a variety of reasons, including societal taboos, personal values and beliefs, past experiences, and preferences. In order to make sure that partners are on the same page, it is necessary to open up communication channels so they can talk about their sexual health needs, expectations, and restrictions.

Partners must be aware of their own and their partner's sexual health in order to negotiate sexual issues in relationships. Sexual health has several facets, including emotional, psychological, and physical health. For any unintended repercussions to be avoided, it is crucial that partners are aware of these facets. For instance, understanding and controlling reproductive health can help prevent infections, while being informed of STD transmission techniques, prevention, and treatment can help reduce infections.

Open communication is the first step in navigating sexual health in relationships. Partners must be willing to communicate any worries or questions they may have and feel at ease discussing sexual health-related issues. Mutual trust, respect, and understanding—three essential elements of any successful relationship—can help you achieve this. Additionally, partners should be open to hearing each other out and offering emotional support as required. Knowing each other's sexual history, including prior sexual behaviors, experiences, and any current sexual health issues, can help improve communication.

Use condoms consistently and appropriately to stop the spread of STDs and unintended pregnancies. Condoms are a crucial component of sexual health. However, wearing condoms can be a touchy subject for some couples, particularly if they are engaged. Couples should be aware that condoms can be used to increase pleasure and solidify their physical link in addition to serving as a means of protection. Therefore, it is crucial to have a conversation about condom use before having sex so that both partners are aware of and at ease with one another's preferences.

Setting sexual boundaries is also crucial for maintaining one's sexual health in relationships. To prevent scenarios when one partner might feel uncomfortable or violated, partners should have a clear awareness of each other's sexual preferences and limits. This can be accomplished by respecting each other's sexual preferences and maintaining open lines of communication and sexual boundaries. To make sure that both parties feel comfortable and are on the same page, this may involve talking about sexual fantasies or preferences.

Another crucial component of sexual health that needs to take priority in relationships is personal hygiene. Both partners should practice proper hygiene, which includes taking regular showers and washing their hands and genitalia both before and after sex. In addition to preventing diseases, this encourages intimacy and increases sexual pleasure.

Along with the aforementioned, consent is necessary for every sexual conduct. Before participating in any sexual activity, partners should show respect for each other's limits and obtain permission. Not only should consent be obtained at the beginning of the sexual activity, but it should also be reiterated throughout. This fosters mutual respect and trust, two essential elements of a healthy partnership.

Another vital component of sexual health that should be given priority in relationships is reproductive health. Couples should talk about their choices for fertility, such as family planning and avoiding unintended pregnancies. Contraceptives like birth control pills, condoms, or other hormonal methods can be used to do this.

In the end, managing sexual health in relationships is a lifelong journey that calls for honest conversation, shared trust, and respect. Given its significance to overall health and well-being, sexual health should be given the attention it merits. Together, partners should endeavor to meet one other's needs and expectations in terms of sexual health, and by clear communication and mutual respect, they may overcome any difficulties that may come up.

CONCLUSION

As a vital component of general well-being, sexual health must be given top priority. The physical and mental health of a person can be significantly impacted by taking proactive steps to preserve sexual health, such as engaging in safe sex and having frequent screenings. People can lead happier and happier lives by recognizing the significance of sexual health and taking appropriate action. In order to dispel the stigma associated with these subjects and make sure that everyone has access to the tools and knowledge they need to maintain their health, it is crucial to discuss sexual health openly with healthcare experts, romantic partners, and family members.

www.ingramcontent.com/pod-product-compliance
Lightning Source LLC
Chambersburg PA
CBHW072343270726
48659CB00023B/2331